Essential Heroes and Fredrick Frankincense

By Caleb Selby

Illustrated by Fenny Fu

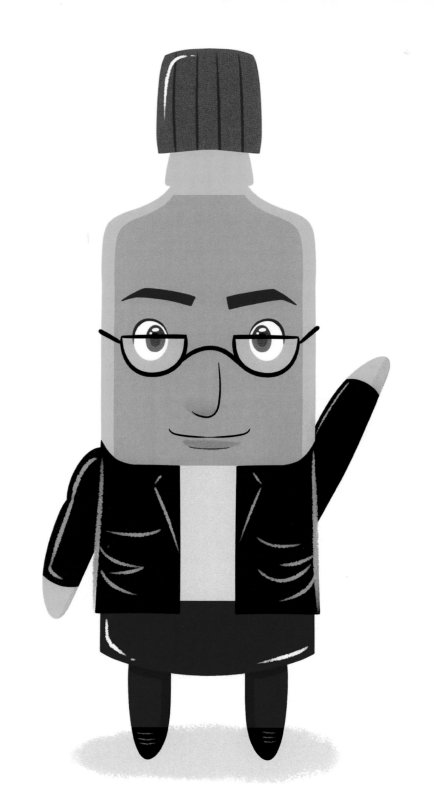

This is Fredrick Frankincense!

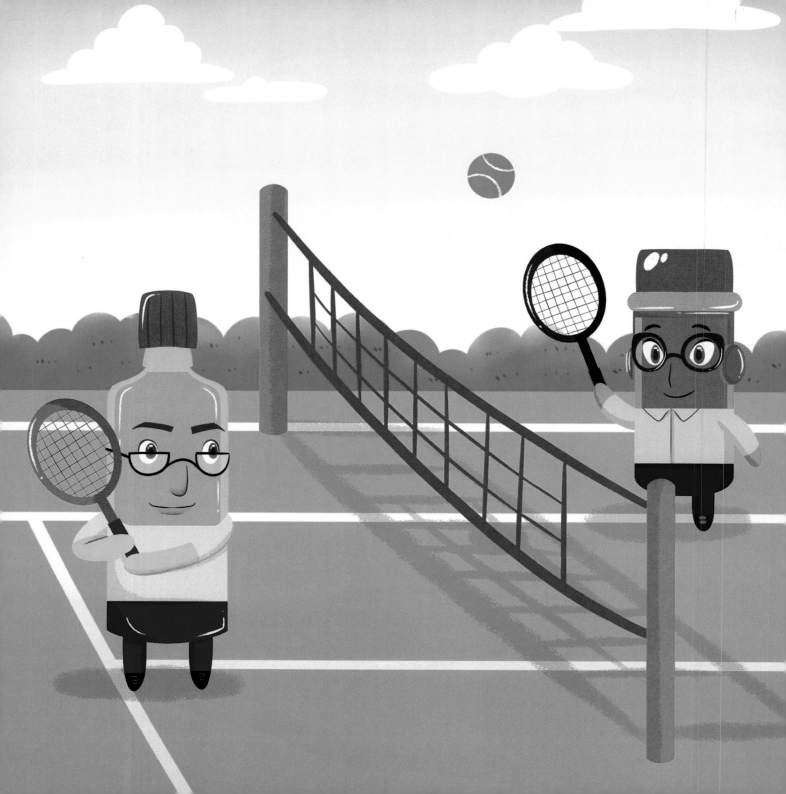

Fredrick Frankincense is strong and determined. He enjoys running, working out, and playing tennis with his friends.

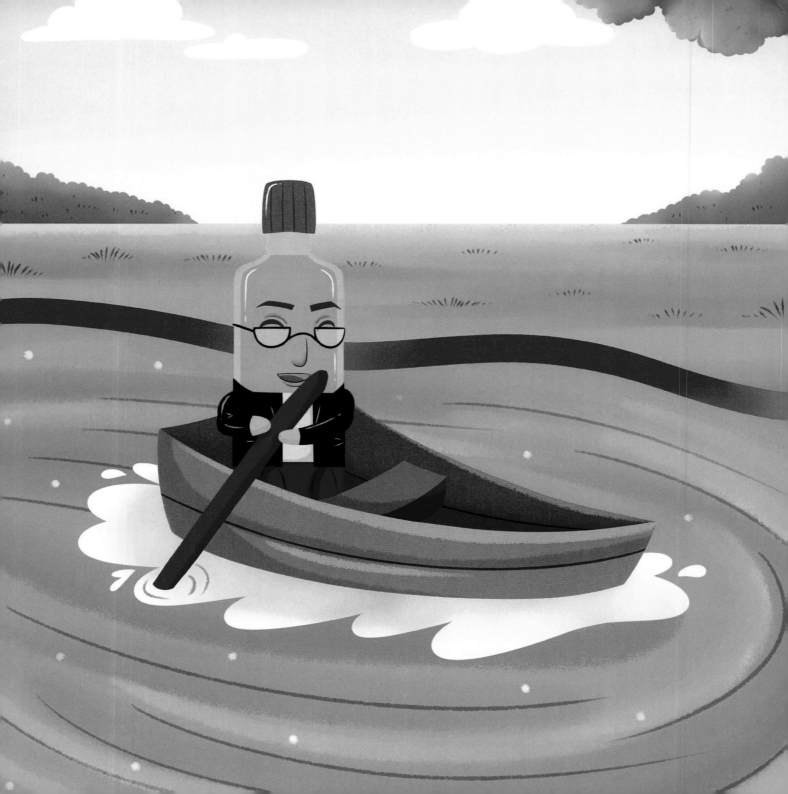

When he is not working out or playing tennis with his friends, Fredrick enjoys boating on the lake. Boating helps Fredrick build strong muscles.

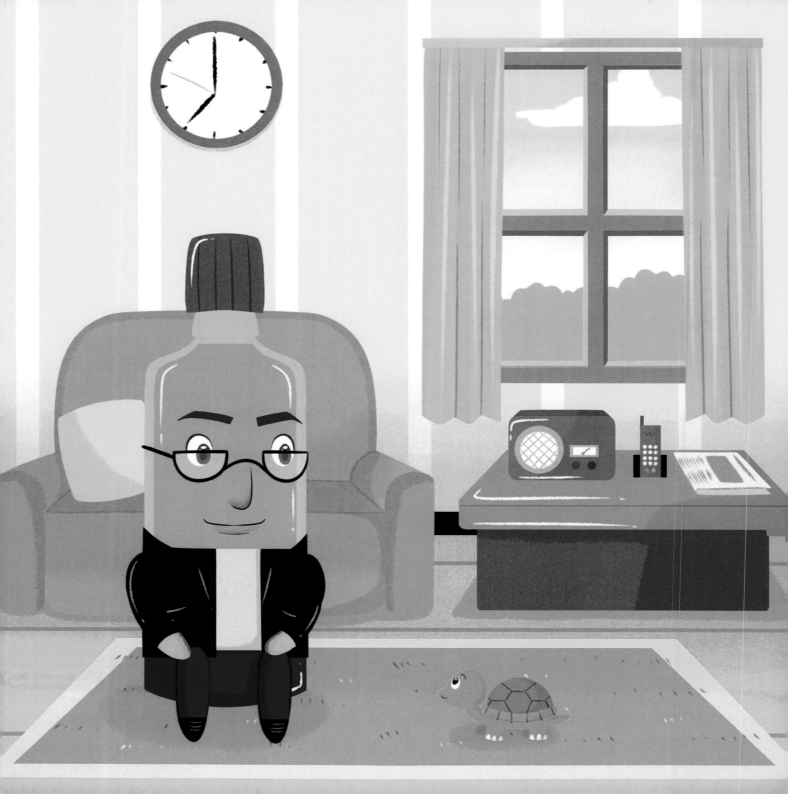

Fredrick lives in a small apartment in Bodyville with his pet turtle named Felicity.

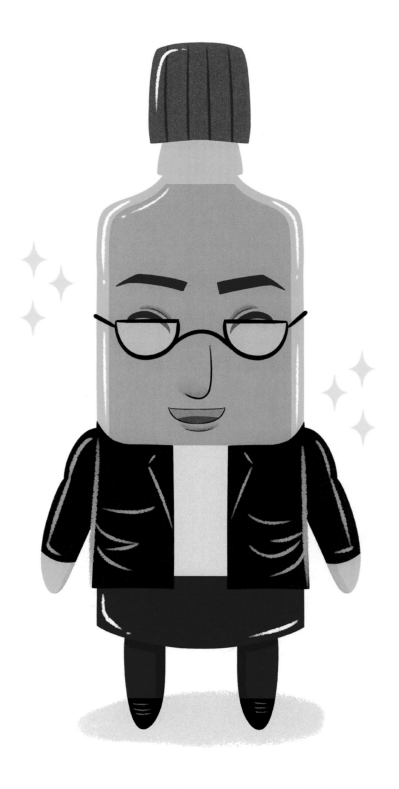

Everyone loves Fredrick. He is a great friend, an excellent tennis player, and he is strong enough to help his friends move their couches and other heavy things.

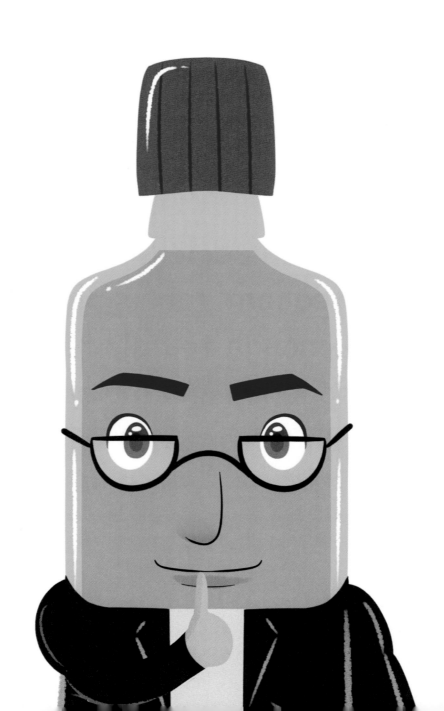

But there is something about Fredrick
that not everyone knows...

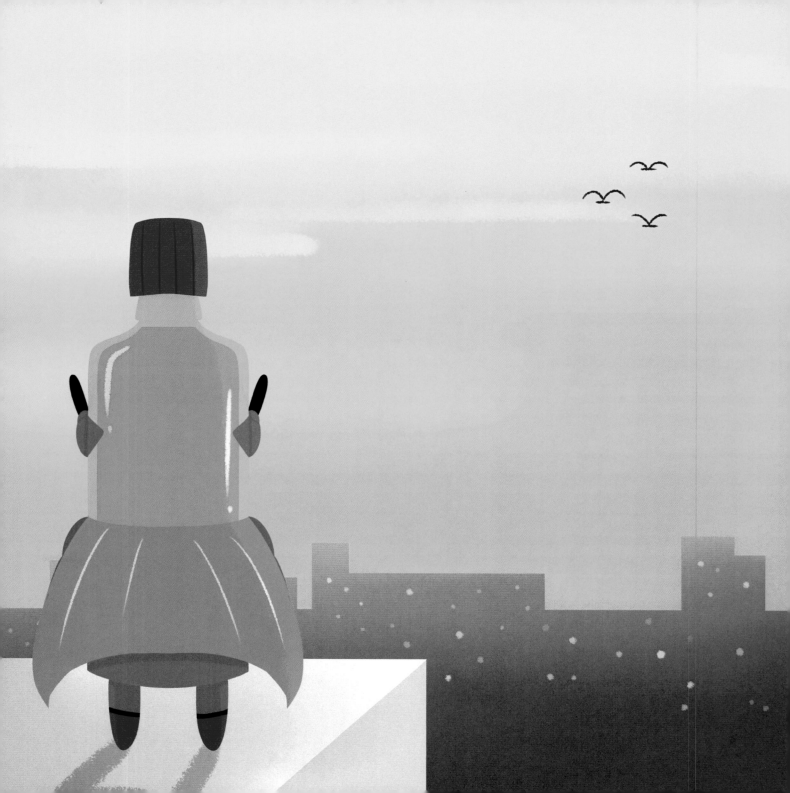

When he is not spending time working out, playing tennis, boating on the lake, or caring for his turtle, Fredrick works for...

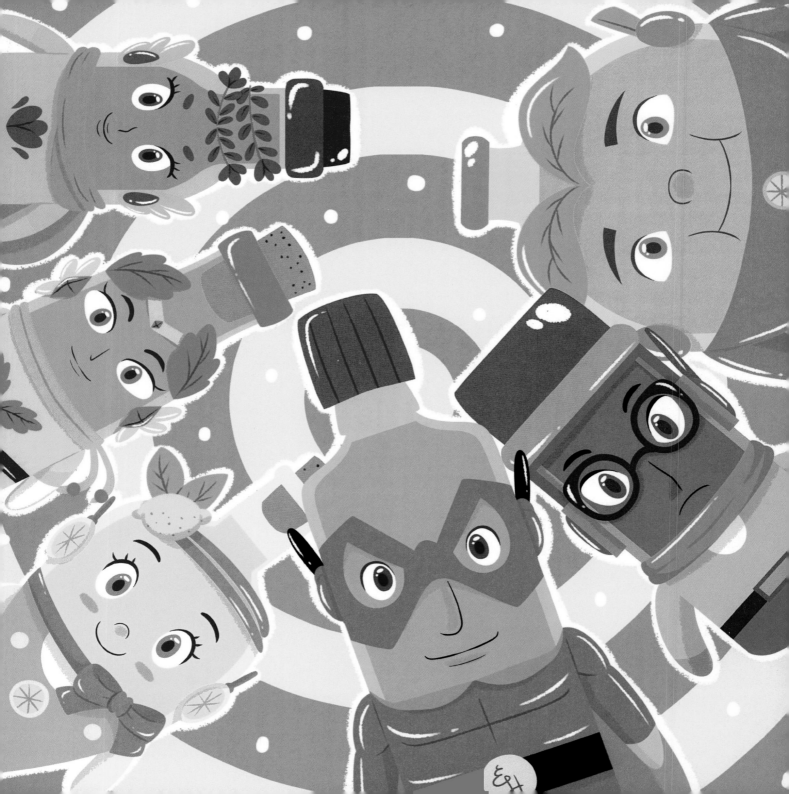

The Essential Heroes!!!

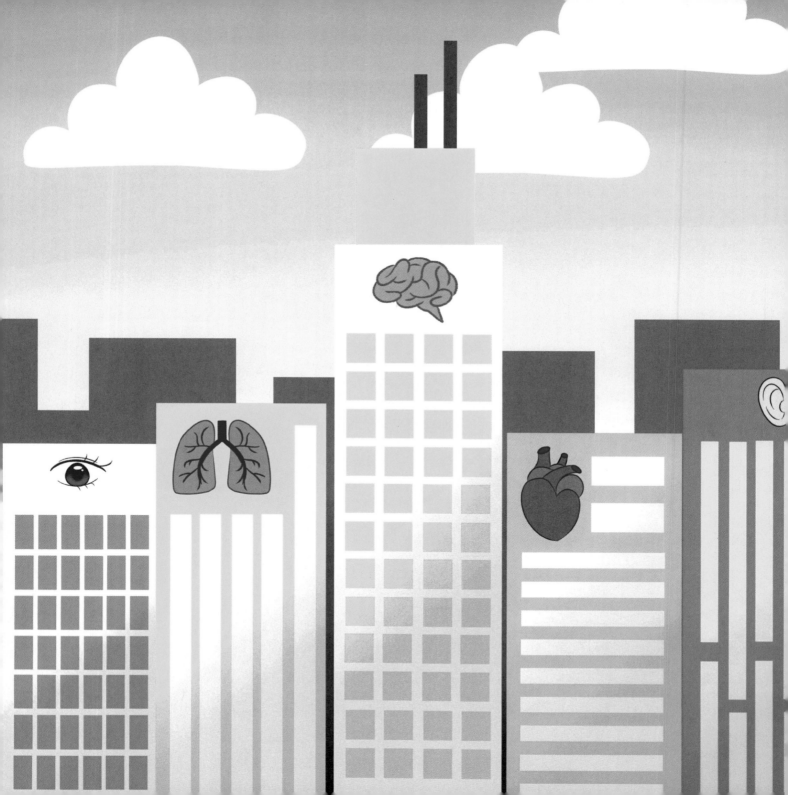

The Essential Heroes are a dedicated team of powerful friends that support Bodyville whenever there is a need!

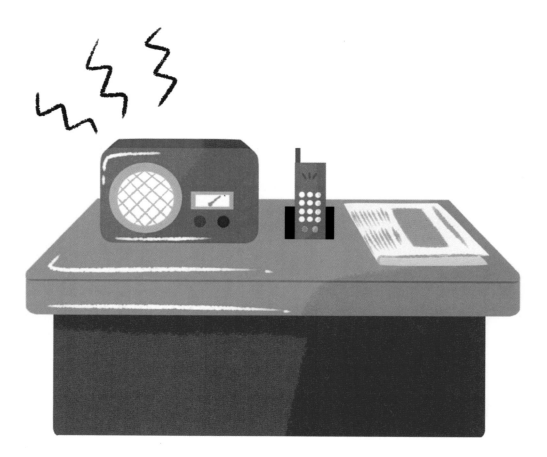

The Essential Heroes are called into action by Mr. Hypo. Mr. Hypo is the allusive and secret leader of the Essential Heroes. Mr. Hypo constantly watches over Bodyville, searching for anything and everything that needs hero help!

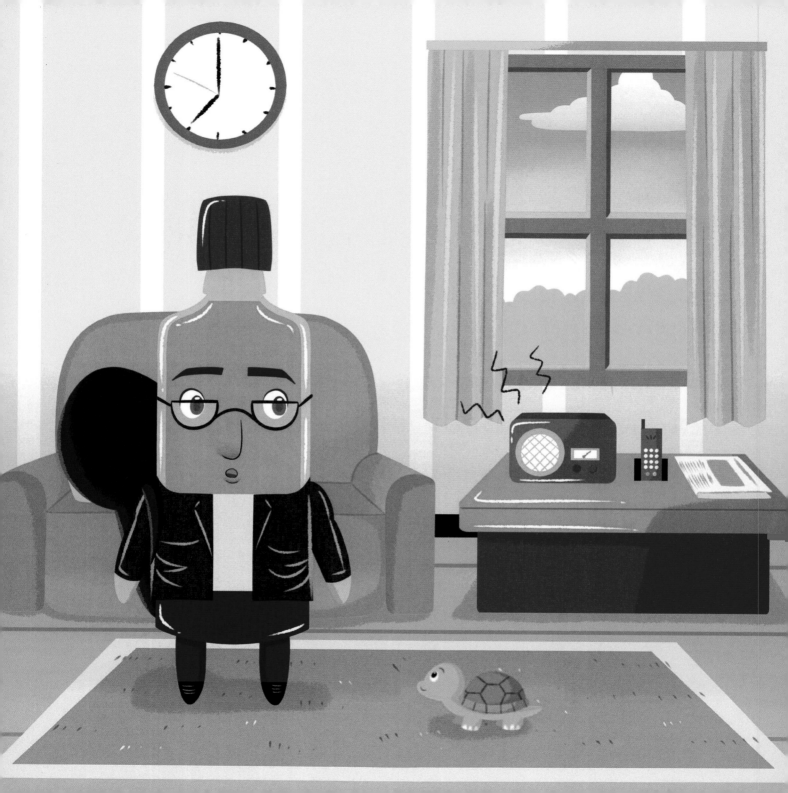

One day, Frederick came home from tennis early because rain clouds had set in above the courts. It was a good thing he was home because just as he walked in, his super secret radio crackled to life.

"This is Hypo calling Fredrick Frankincense! I repeat, this is Hypo calling Fredrick Frankincense! Come in Fredrick!"

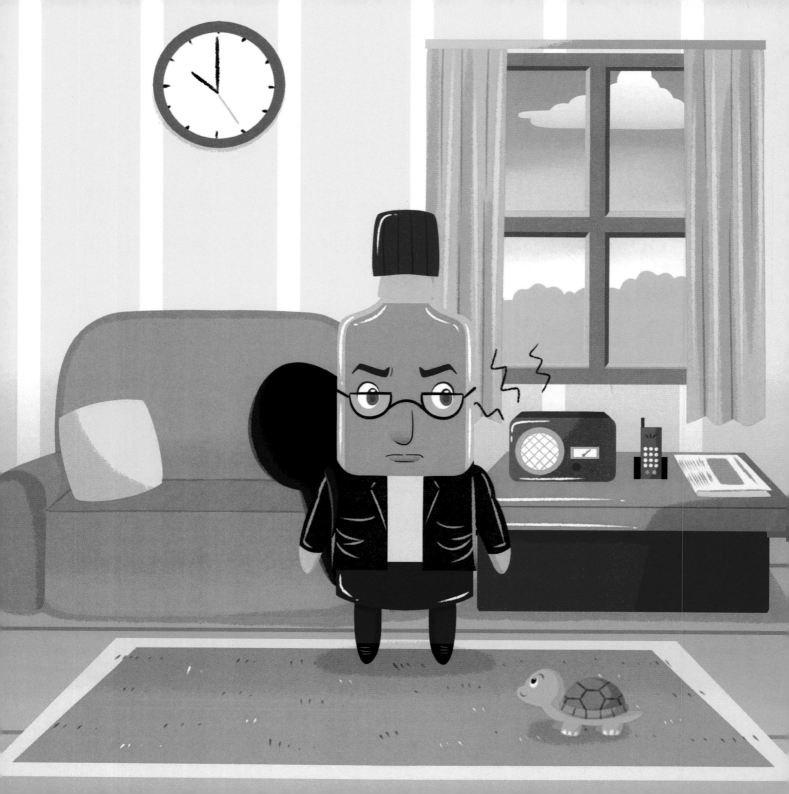

"Fredrick Frankincense here! Go ahead Mr. Hypo!" Fredrick answered quickly.

"I'm so glad you're home!" Mr. Hypo said, his voice sounding frazzled. "We just received word that the Horrible Hoard has been spotted downtown!"

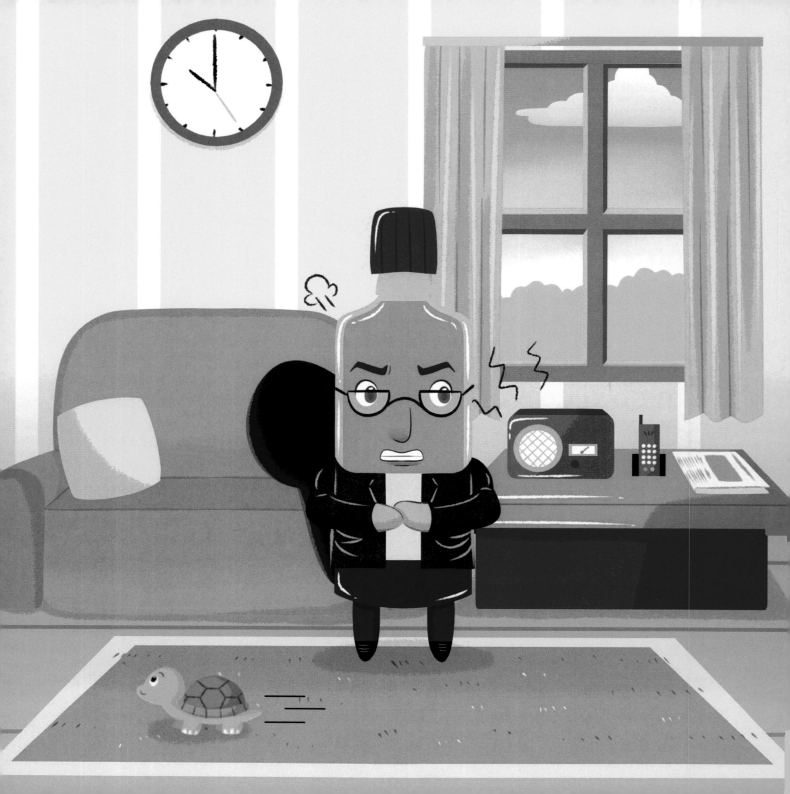

"Those dastardly devils!" Fredrick shouted angrily, scaring Felicity who scampered out of the room as fast as she could go, which wasn't very fast.

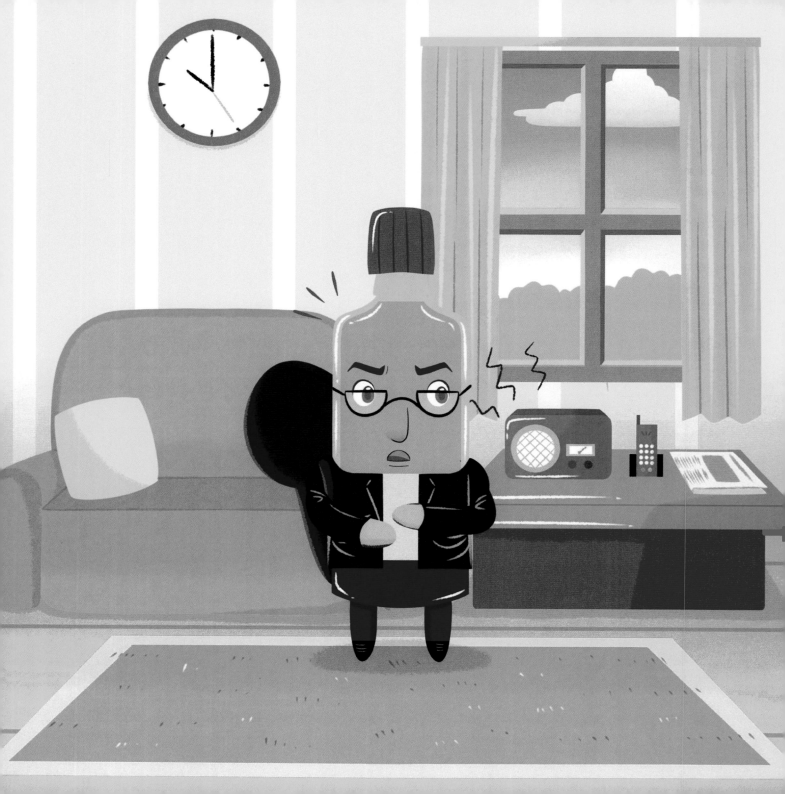

"My sources tell me that they are planning on causing havoc at the cerebral tower sometime tonight," Hypo continued. "Can you stop them?"

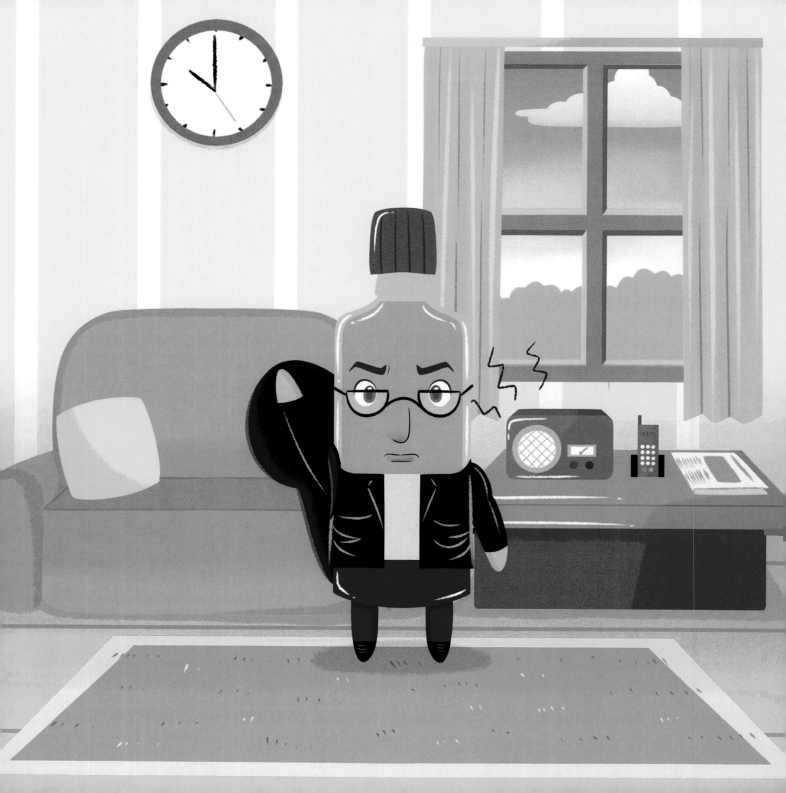

"I have no choice but to try!" Fredrick shouted out confidently. "We must maintain the Bodyville systems, at all costs!"

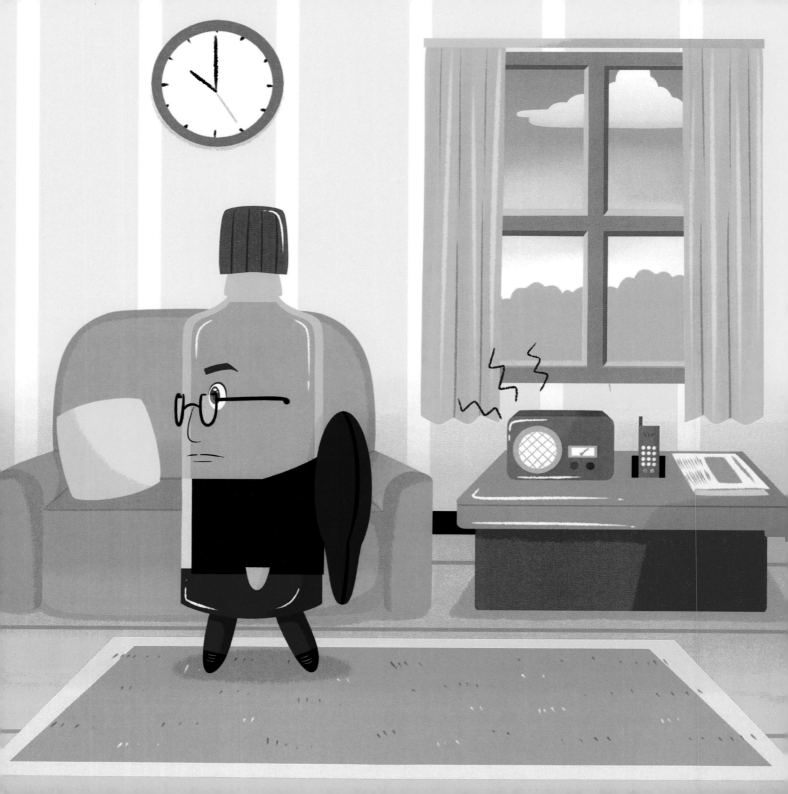

"Then hurry!" said Mr. Hypo forcefully as Fredrick walked out of the room. "There is no time for delay! You know how much damage the Horrible Hoard can cause!"

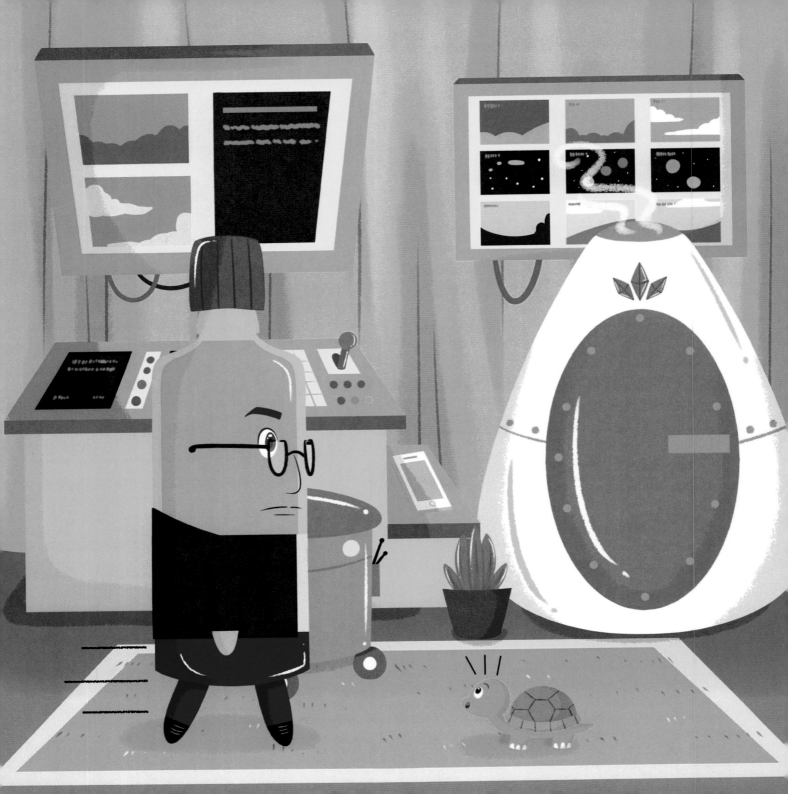

Fredrick startled Felicity when he burst into his diffuser room.

"Sorry Felicity," he said as he briskly walked passed her. "Bodyville needs me. I'll be back tonight."

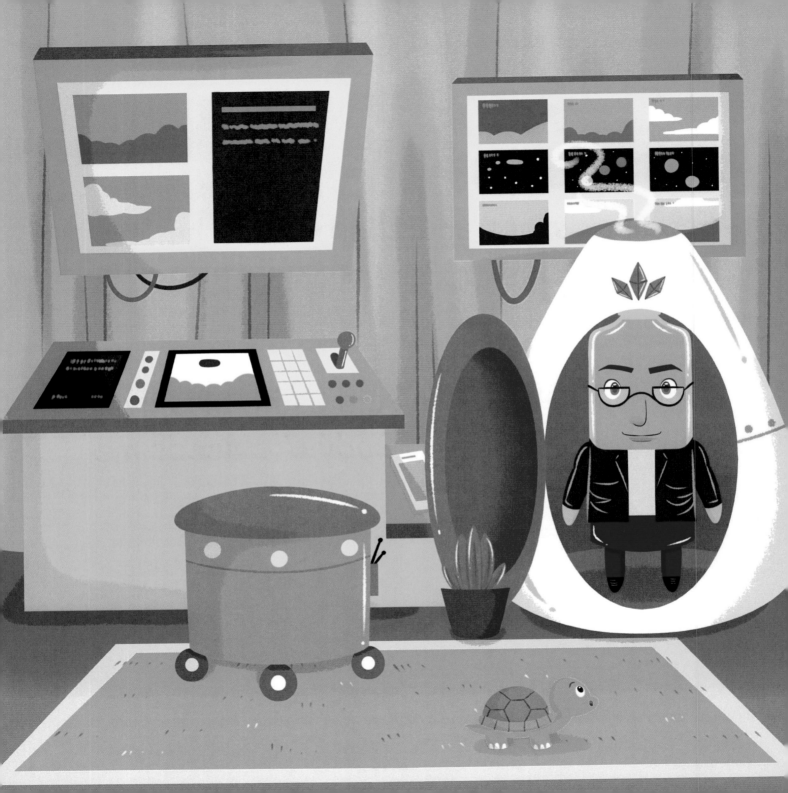

Fredrick stepped into the diffuser, breathed in deeply, and then closed the door. He was ready for action!

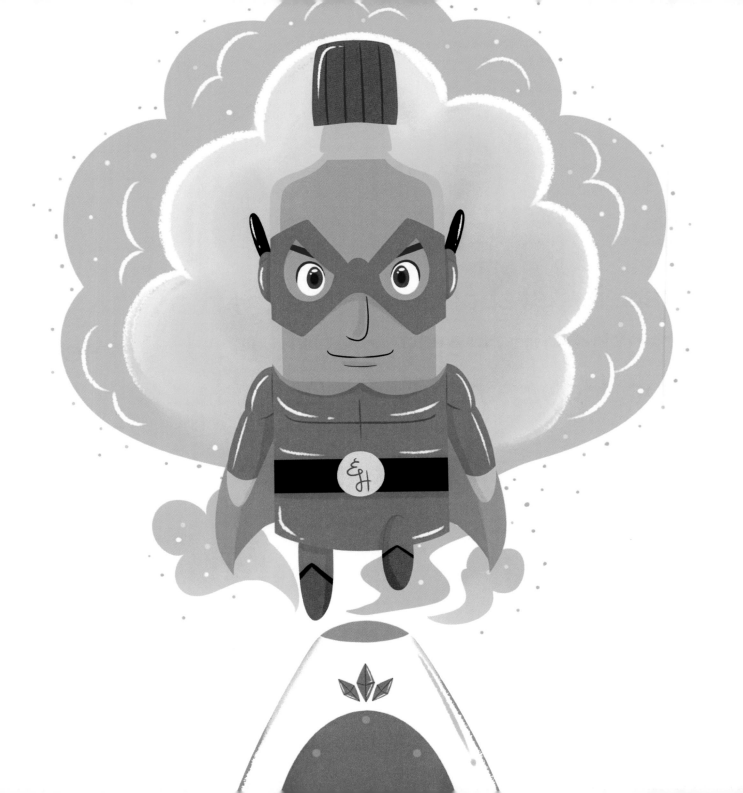

Fredrick emerged from the diffuser as Fredrick Frankincense! Now he was ready to support Bodyville!

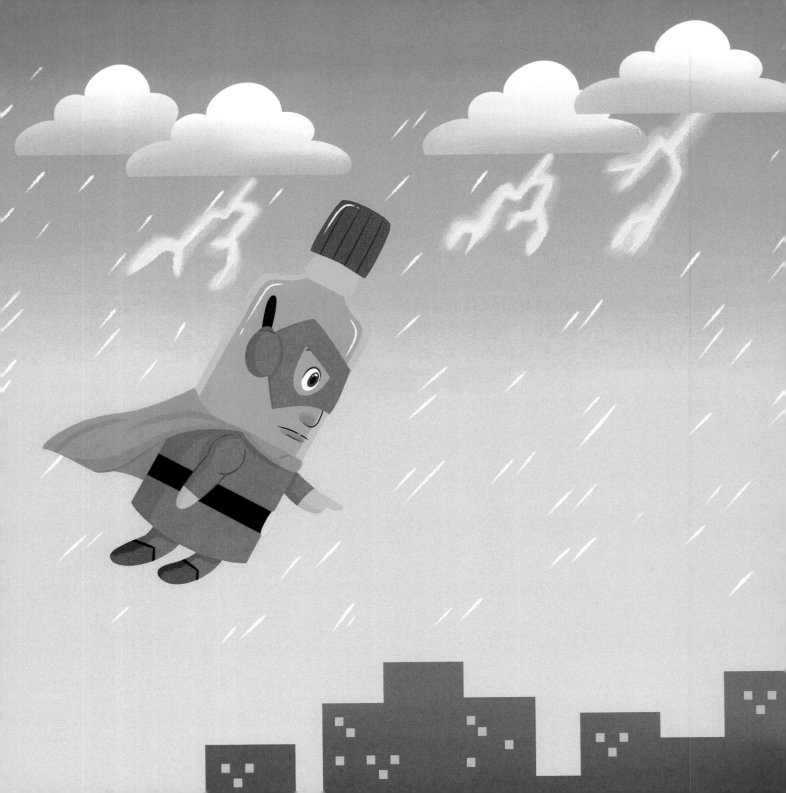

The dark clouds that ended his tennis match, had now begun to rain. Loud claps of thunder and flashes of lightning added to the dreary scene. Fredrick paid the storm no heed. He was on a mission and nothing was going to stop him from completing it.

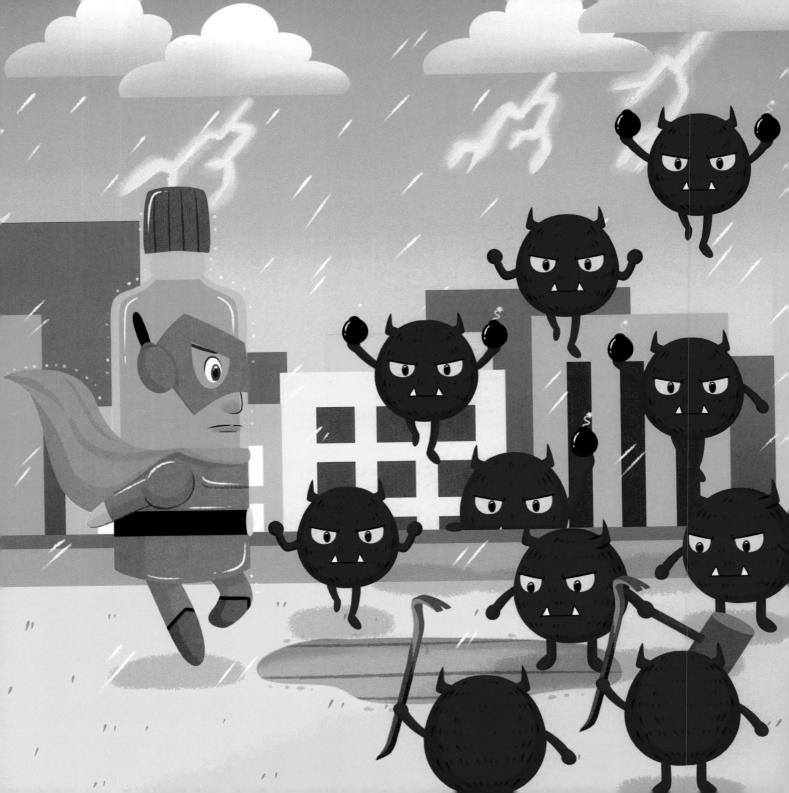

Fredrick found the Horrible Hoard quickly, thanks, in part, to the lightning flashes that illuminated them in the darkness.

As Fredrick landed, the Horrible Hoard looked as if they were living up to their name. They were armed for destruction with crowbars, hammers, and little bombs. Fredrick knew he had to act quickly!

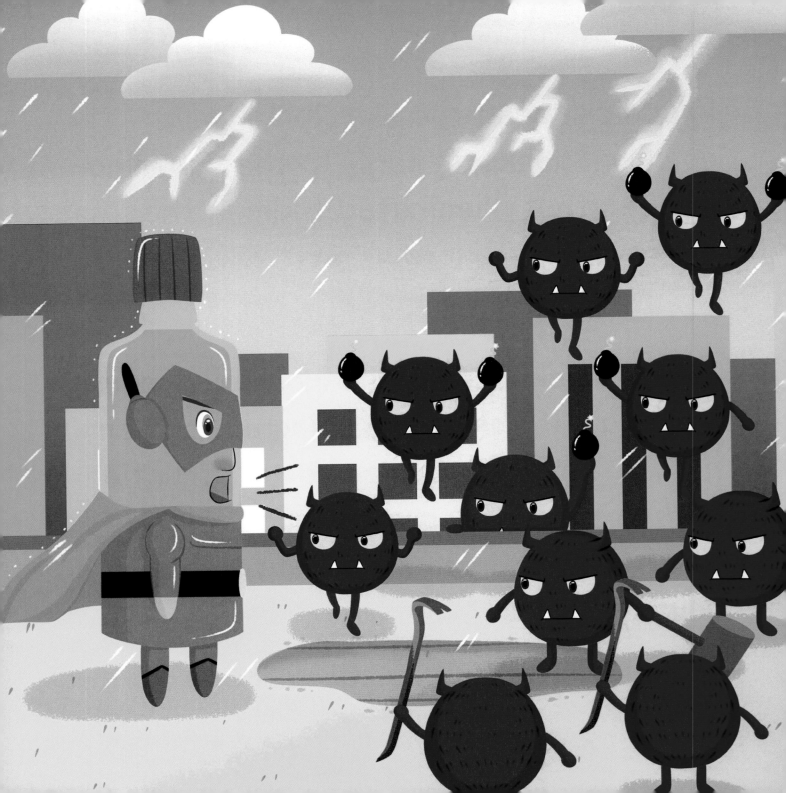

"Leave Bodyville alone!" yelled Fredrick as the Horrible Hoard looked at him angrily.

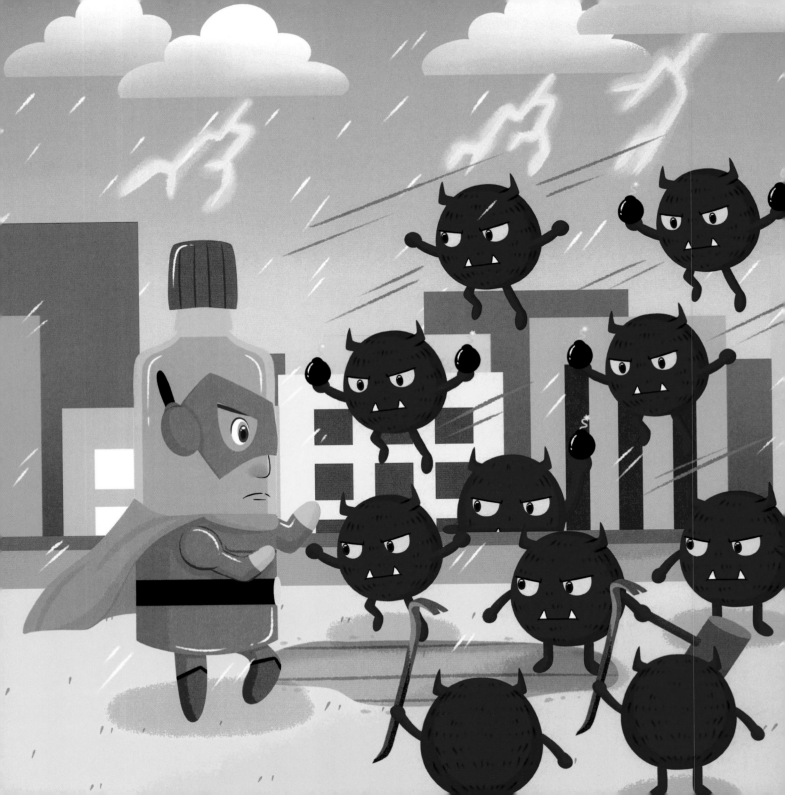

Without a word, the Horrible Hoard lunged at Fredrick. Fredrick put up his hands to fight them off, but there were just too many.

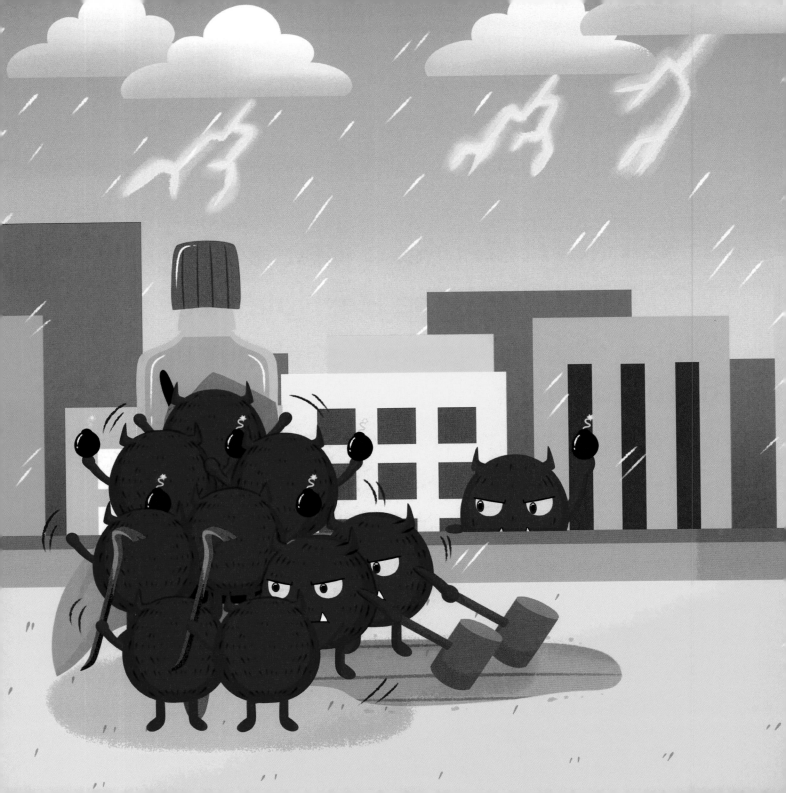

The Hoard piled onto Fredrick, who couldn't push them off fast enough. Things were looking grim for the Essential Hero.

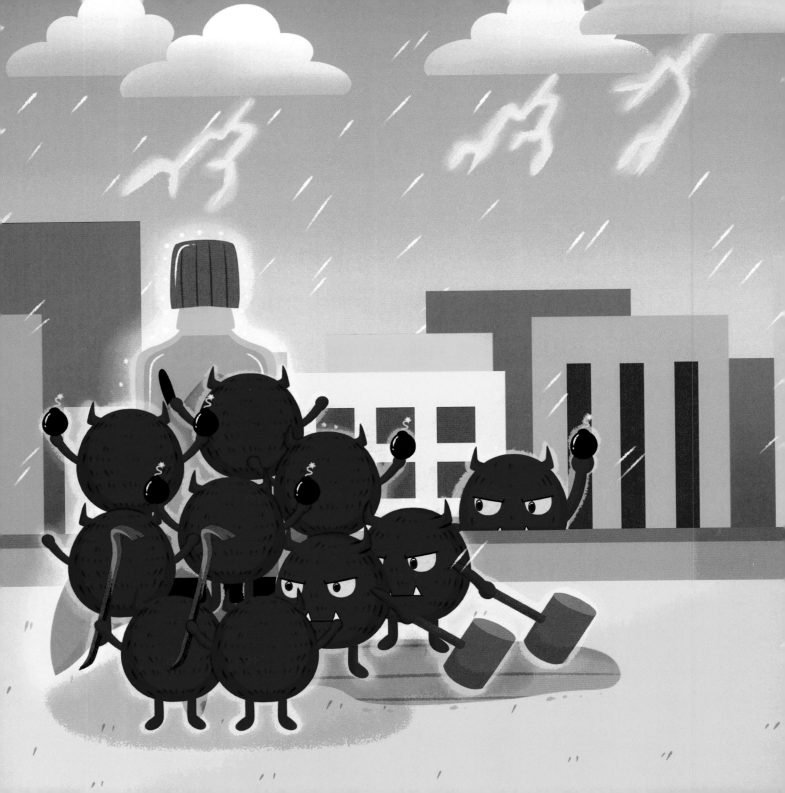

But just as all hope seemed lost for poor Fredrick, his power began to pulse outward. It started low and soft at first but slowly built up until...

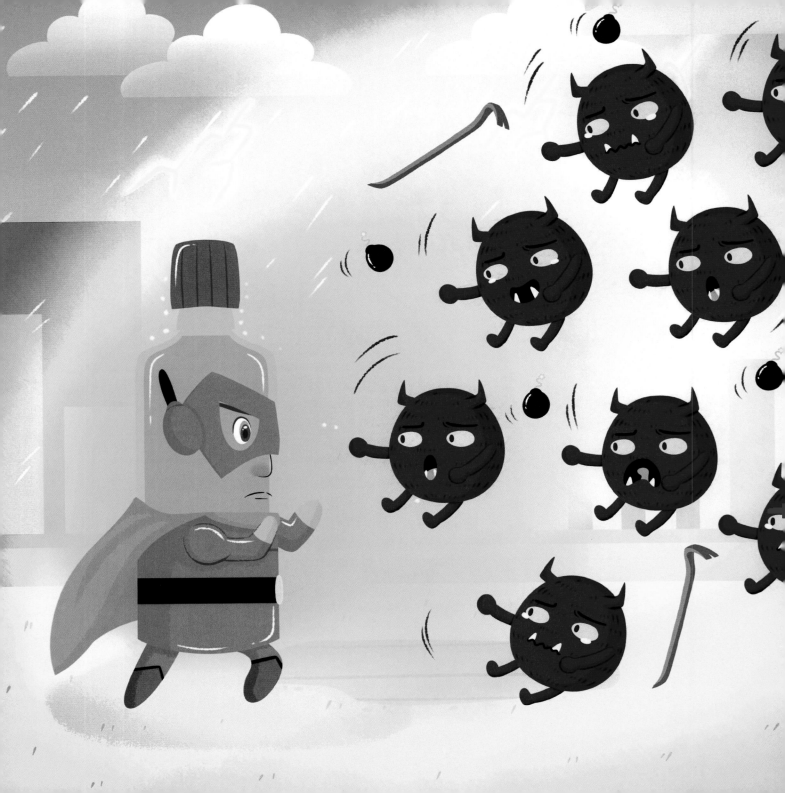

"Wham!" he erupted in a powerful wave of reddish light that sent the Horrible Hoard flying backwards.

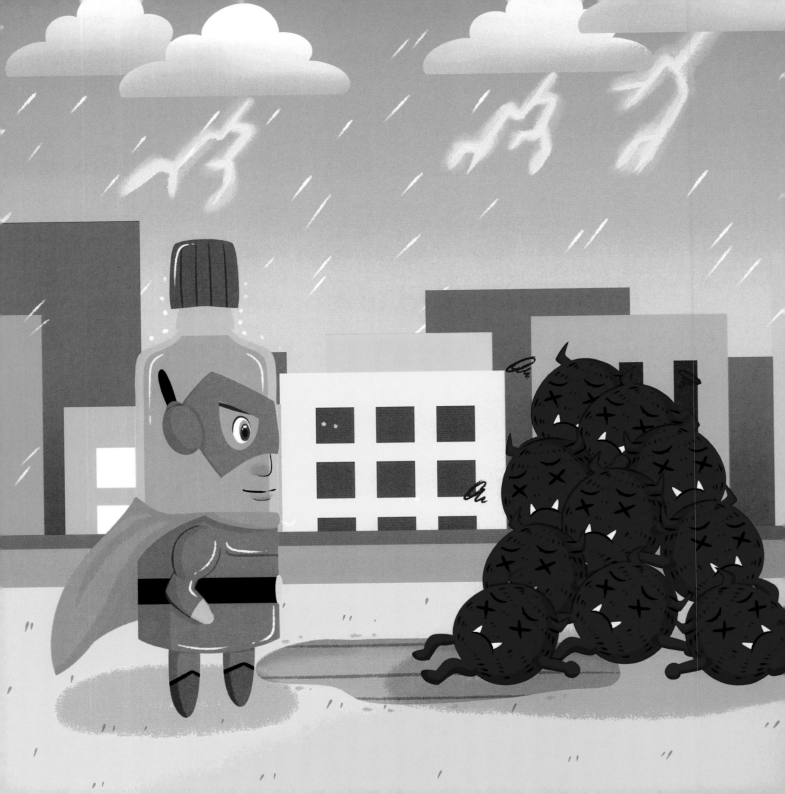

The Hoard ended up in a giant heap, their heads spinning after recovering from the amazing power of Fredrick Frankincense.

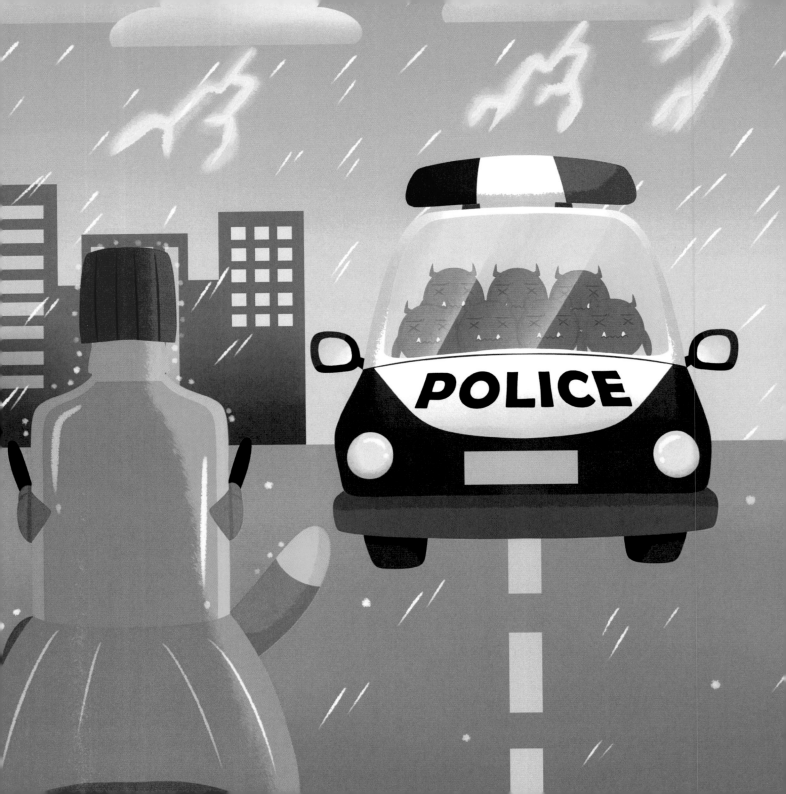

Fredrick waved goodbye as the Horrible Hoard was packed into a police car and driven away to the Bodyville jail.

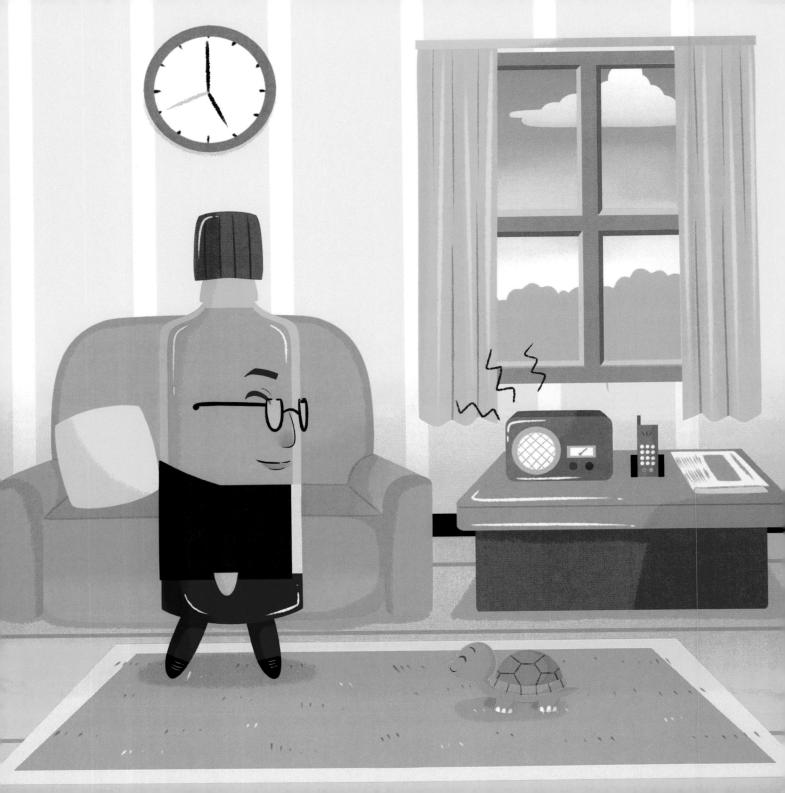

Felicity beamed with happiness when Fredrick walked back into the house.

"Nice job out there tonight!" Hypo called from the radio, as Fredrick walked past with a satisfied smile on his face.

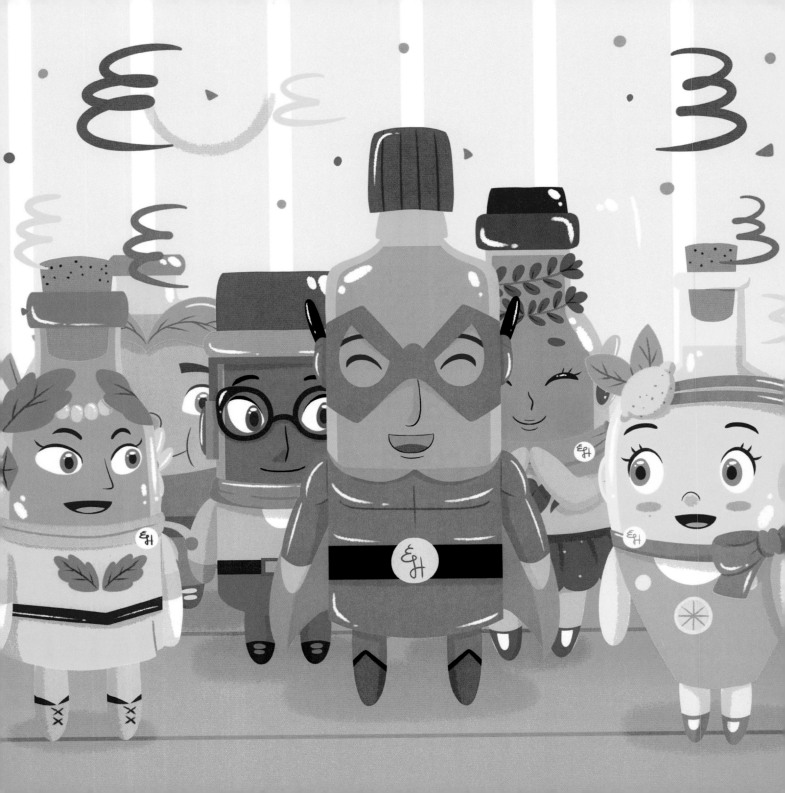

Hooray for Fredrick Frankincense! He is a great member of the Essential Heroes team!